NAVIGATING EWING SARCOMA WITH CONFIDENCE AND CARE

Mastering The Journey And Empowering Strategies For Quick Approach To Cancer Recovery With Assurance And Compassion

DR. WESLEY IAN

DISCLAIMER

The information in this book is not meant to replace professional medical advice, diagnosis, or treatment; rather, it is meant mainly for general informational reasons. If you have any questions about a medical problem, you should always consult your doctor or another trained health expert. Don't ever discount expert medical advice or put off getting it because of something you've read in this book.

Any negative effects or repercussions arising from the usage of the material provided herein are not the responsibility of the book's author or publisher. It should be noted by readers that the material in this book is not all-inclusive and might not address every facet of the subject. Furthermore, new research may have an impact on how health concerns are understood or treated because medical knowledge is always changing.

No particular test, treatment, method, or product mentioned in this book is endorsed or promoted by the author or publisher. The reader assumes all risk associated with using the information included in this book.

Before making any big decisions regarding your health, it's crucial to speak with a licensed healthcare provider. The relationship between a patient and their healthcare practitioner should not be replaced by this book, nor is it meant to offer medical advice.

The opinions presented in this book are the author's and may not necessarily represent those of the publisher. Any errors, omissions, or inaccuracies in the information in this book are not the responsibility of the author or publisher.

It is recommended that readers independently confirm any information contained in this book and speak with a healthcare provider about their specific medical needs and state of health.

TABLE OF CONTENTS

ABOUT THE BOOK

Navigating Ewing Sarcoma with Confidence and Care is a useful resource for individuals and families confronting the challenges of Ewing sarcoma, a rare and frequently complex form of cancer. The book is expertly written and offers a thorough guide that addresses the emotional, social, and practical aspects of navigating this trip in addition to medical reasons.

By introducing the book and stating its goal, the introduction establishes the mood for the reader. It highlights how crucial it is to manage Ewing sarcoma with caution and confidence while appreciating how complex the process is. This method lays the groundwork for the next chapters, which focus on different aspects of the voyage.

The groundwork "Understanding Ewing Sarcoma," which defines the illness, examines its etiology and risk factors, and describes the diagnostic and staging procedures. This knowledge is essential for enabling people to appreciate the complexity of their illness and promoting well-informed decision-making.

This book provides a comprehensive analysis of the therapeutic landscape, including the multidisciplinary approach, surgical possibilities, radiation therapy, chemotherapy regimes, and new developments in treatment modalities. By providing readers with a thorough awareness of all of the possibilities, this overview empowers them to take an active role in choosing their course of therapy.

In this book, "Building a Support System," the significance of having a strong support system—which includes friends, family, and support groups—is discussed. It covers practical issues as well as patients' emotional and mental health, offering direction on how to find resources for all-encompassing help.

The complexity of treatment options, efficient communication with healthcare providers, getting second opinions, and controlling adverse effects of therapy are all covered in "Navigating Medical Decisions," This section gives people the tools they need to take an active role in their healthcare journey while also building confidence and a sense of control.

The book delves deeper into life during treatment and offers helpful tips on how to deal with day-to-day obstacles, dietary concerns, exercise, and integrative therapies. It acknowledges the significance of attending to the overall health and welfare of patients while they are receiving therapy.

The perspectives on survivorship, long-term issues, and the need for activism and empowerment are expanded upon in this book "Looking to the Future," offers information on new developments in the study of Ewing sarcoma, possible therapies, and the critical role that advocacy will play in determining the course of the illness.

Navigating Ewing Sarcoma with Confidence and Care is an invaluable resource that offers a comprehensive strategy to empower people with Ewing sarcoma and their support systems, going beyond the clinical aspects of the illness. This book offers a thorough road map for negotiating the intricacies of Ewing sarcoma with assurance and compassion through a careful examination of medical, emotional, and advocacy-related subjects.

CHAPTER ONE

THE INTRODUCTION TO EWING SARCOMA

COMPREHENDING EWING SARCOMA

Ewing Sarcoma is an uncommon and very aggressive kind of cancer that mostly affects soft tissues and bones, especially in young adults and children. Ewing Sarcoma is named after the American pathologist James Ewing, who originally identified the illness in the early 20th century. Diagnosing, treating, and managing Ewing Sarcoma presents several difficulties. The purpose of this introduction is to examine the basic ideas related to Ewing Sarcoma, including its definition, etiology, risk factors, diagnosis techniques, staging, and typical symptoms.

WHAT IS SARCOMA EWING?

Ewing Sarcoma is a kind of cancer that develops in the soft tissues or bones and is distinguished by aberrant cell proliferation. While it can happen to anyone at any age, children and teenagers are the ones who are diagnosed with it the most frequently. Although it can also affect other places like the pelvis, chest wall, and spine, the tumor most commonly appears in the long bones, such as the arms and legs. Ewing Sarcoma is a member of the larger group of cancers referred to as Ewing Sarcoma Family cancers (ESFT), which are comparable in terms of cellular properties and genetic abnormalities.

REASONS AND DANGER FACTORS:

Although the exact cause of Ewing Sarcoma is yet unknown, genetic changes are thought to be the cause. Scientists have discovered a particular genetic translocation that involves chromosomes 11 and 22 and causes the FLI1 and EWSR1 genes to fuse. This fusion is a characteristic feature of Ewing Sarcoma and is essential to the pathogenesis of the illness. A higher risk of getting Ewing Sarcoma has been linked to several risk factors, even though the precise causes of these genetic alterations remain unclear.

These variables include exposure to ionizing radiation, specific genetic disorders, and a family history of cancer.

IDENTIFICATION AND STAGE

A combination of laboratory testing, biopsy techniques and medical imaging is used to diagnose Ewing Sarcoma. Imaging modalities such as MRIs, CTs, X-rays, and bone scans are frequently used to see the tumor and determine its size. However, a biopsy—which involves taking a sample of the tumor tissue and examining it under a microscope—is necessary to provide a definitive diagnosis.

Molecular tests and immunohistochemistry might also be used to verify whether the distinctive genetic translocation is present. Determining the degree of the disease's dissemination requires staging, which frequently entails a mix of imaging tests and perhaps surgical exploration. Creating a suitable treatment strategy and determining the prognosis is made easier by the staging process.

TYPICAL SYMPTOMS

Numerous symptoms can indicate Ewing Sarcoma, albeit they can change based on the tumor's size and location. Ewing Sarcoma is characterized by chronic discomfort and swelling in the afflicted soft tissue or bone. People may also have fever, exhaustion, and weight loss. As the tumor enlarges, it may press against nearby structures, causing problems and functional impairments. For a timely diagnosis and course of treatment, early detection of these symptoms is essential.

Conclusively, Ewing Sarcoma is a powerful foe in the field of pediatric and adolescent cancers, requiring a thorough comprehension of its characteristics, etiology, diagnostic techniques, staging, and typical symptoms. To lay the groundwork for a more thorough examination of the difficulties and developments in the treatment of Ewing sarcoma, this introduction offers a basic summary of the main ideas related to the condition.

CHAPTER TWO

THE LANDSCAPE OF TREATMENT

MULTIDISCIPLINARY METHOD

A multidisciplinary approach has become essential in the ever-changing field of medical therapy to effectively manage complex health issues. Using a multidisciplinary approach, several medical specialists work together to create a customized treatment plan that takes into account all of the different facets of a patient's health. This method is especially useful when treating diseases like cancer, as a group of doctors, nurses, radiologists, and other medical specialists work together to provide a comprehensive and efficient treatment plan.

OPTIONS FOR SURGERY

Surgery is a key element of the therapeutic paradigm, providing a variety of alternatives to treat different ailments. Tumor excision, tissue healing, and the relief of various clinical diseases are the goals of surgical operations. The location and stage of the disease, the patient's general health, and the likelihood of a full recovery after surgery all play a role in the surgical treatment that is chosen. Technological developments in surgery have improved the accuracy and effectiveness of surgical operations, reducing patient discomfort and hastening recovery. Examples of these developments include robotic-assisted surgery and minimally invasive procedures.

CHEMOTHERAPY PROCEDURES

Chemotherapy is an essential systemic treatment for cancer and several other disorders. As part of chemotherapy treatments, strong medications that target quickly dividing cells—including cancer cells—are administered. Chemotherapy regimens are meticulously customized by the multidisciplinary team according to the particular form of cancer, its stage, and the health profile of each patient. Even though side effects from chemotherapy are common, research is currently being conducted to provide tailored therapies that maximize benefits and minimize negative effects, leading to the emergence of customized medicine.

RADIATION TREATMENT

Another essential component of cancer treatment is radiation therapy, which uses strong radiation doses to kill or harm cancer cells. This targeted method is used in conjunction with surgery or chemotherapy to treat particular tumors or diseased areas. Proton therapy and intensity-modulated radiation therapy (IMRT) are two examples of technological innovations that allow for more accurate targeting of cancer cells while protecting surrounding healthy tissues. The incorporation of imaging technologies enhances treatment planning and guarantees the best possible therapeutic results.

NEW APPROACHES TO TREATMENT

Emerging therapy techniques constantly change the treatment landscape as medical research progresses. For example, immunotherapy uses the body's immune system to identify and eliminate cancer cells. This novel method of cancer treatment represents a paradigm change and shows promise for treating a range of cancers. Additionally, targeted medicines, molecular profiling, and gene therapies are at the forefront of precision medicine, personalizing interventions based on the unique genetic composition of each patient's disease. These changing approaches highlight how dynamic the therapeutic environment is and present fresh opportunities to enhance patient outcomes and quality of life.

A multidisciplinary strategy that acknowledges the complex interactions between different medical specializations in creating complete and customized interventions characterizes the treatment landscape. Radiation therapy, chemotherapy, and surgery continue to be mainstays in the treatment regimen, each improving with new scientific and technological discoveries.

CHAPTER THREE

ESTABLISHING A NETWORK OF SUPPORT

THE IMPORTANCE OF FRIENDS AND FAMILY

Creating a strong support network is essential for overcoming obstacles in life and preserving general well-being. The ties to family and friends form the foundation of this support system. These relationships are essential for giving people emotional support, comprehension, and a feeling of community. Family members can be a dependable source of support during trying times because of their innate closeness and shared past. Selecting friends based on compatibility and shared ideals adds another level of support by providing a variety of viewpoints and occasionally a more impartial one. Friends and family work together to create a vital support system that promotes emotional stability and resilience.

GETTING IN TOUCH WITH SUPPORT GROUPS

Apart from intimate connections, joining a support group can greatly improve an individual's capacity to manage a range of life obstacles. Support groups provide a special setting where others with comparable problems can come together to exchange experiences, wisdom, and coping techniques. These support groups offer a sense of connection and understanding that can be crucial in overcoming feelings of isolation, whether one is dealing with health concerns, bereavement, or special life transitions. Being a part of these organizations not only validates personal experiences but also offers a way to learn from the tactics of others and develop a group strength that has the potential to be transformative.

EMOTIONAL AND MENTAL HEALTH

Integral mental and emotional health is the foundation of a complete support network. It entails treating mental health with the same respect and consideration as physical health. Getting professional assistance when required, such as through counseling or therapy, is a proactive move toward preserving mental and emotional equilibrium. In addition to helping with stress and anxiety management, a support network that places a high priority on mental health promotes resilience and personal development in the face of adversity.

REALISTIC ASSISTANCE AND MATERIALS

A comprehensive support system must include resources and helpful assistance. This includes providing concrete aid during hard times, including cash support, daycare, or support with logistics. Having access to pertinent resources—whether via government initiatives, local groups, or internet sites—can reduce pragmatic difficulties and improve a person's general well-being. A support system makes sure that the difficulties encountered are not carried alone by allocating roles and gathering resources, creating a cooperative atmosphere that encourages group problem-solving.

Creating a support system is a complex process that includes fostering deep relationships with family and friends, participating in support groups, placing a high value on one's mental and emotional health, and utilizing available resources and practical help. This network is strong because of its diversity and members' willingness to work together, which creates a strong base for overcoming life's challenges.

CHAPTER FOUR

MAKING MEDICAL DECISIONS

COMPREHENDING AVAILABLE TREATMENTS

Understanding available treatments is a critical first step in making medical decisions. People are frequently presented with a variety of therapy options while dealing with health-related issues, each having its advantages and disadvantages. Patients must be fully informed about all of the alternatives that are open to them, including the type of treatment that will be used, the expected results, any possible adverse effects, and the overall influence on their quality of life. Making decisions that are in line with the patient's values and preferences is made easier with this insight.

INTERACTING WITH HEALTHCARE PROFESSIONALS

Making decisions requires effective communication with healthcare providers. Patients and healthcare providers can work together to build a collaborative connection when honest and open communication is established. It should be encouraged for patients to voice their concerns and desires as well as to seek clarification and ask questions.

To encourage a shared decision-making approach, healthcare providers should also make an effort to clearly and understandably communicate difficult medical facts. Patients are actively involved in the decision-making process and have a thorough grasp of their medical condition and treatment alternatives because of this collaborative communication.

SECOND VIEWS AND METHODS OF MAKING DECISIONS

When making medical decisions, getting a second opinion is a legitimate and frequently advised step. It can offer more information, different viewpoints, and a more thorough comprehension of the options.

In complex or serious medical circumstances, second opinions can be very helpful as they provide patients the chance to consider other techniques and treatment regimens. In the medical field, decision-making techniques should include carefully analyzing all available data, balancing advantages and risks, and matching choices to personal beliefs and objectives. Having conversations with several medical specialists can help ensure that decisions are made with a broader perspective.

TAKING CARE OF SIDE EFFECTS OF TREATMENT

Patients frequently have to consider the potential negative effects of medical treatments while making decisions. Patients must communicate openly and honestly with healthcare providers about any potential negative effects related to a treatment they have chosen. Comprehending the probability and intensity of adverse effects enables patients to make knowledgeable choices and anticipate possible obstacles in advance. In turn, healthcare professionals are essential in controlling and minimizing side effects, offering assistance, and modifying treatment regimens as necessary.

To ensure that people are ready for any obstacles that may come up throughout their chosen therapy, it is essential to take probable side effects into account during the entire decision-making process.

LIVING THROUGH THERAPY AND OVERCOMING DAILY OBSTACLES

Living during treatment presents a wide range of daily obstacles for those managing the intricate world of medical interventions.

Every day might bring different challenges, from the psychological impact of dealing with a medical emergency to the logistical demands of scheduling visits and handling prescription drugs. Patients frequently struggle with the uncertainty surrounding their disease, necessitating a careful balancing act between optimism and pessimism. During this time, coping strategies become extremely important, and support systems are vital in assisting people in navigating the emotional rollercoaster that frequently follows therapy.

NUTRITIONAL CONSIDERATIONS

Managing one's diet is a crucial part of living during treatment. It is impossible to overestimate the effects of different treatments on hunger, digestion, and general nutritional health. Individuals may experience taste alterations, dietary aversions, or trouble eating a balanced diet. In addition to maintaining physical health, nutrition plays a crucial role in boosting immunity and promoting the body's resiliency during medical interventions. Nutritionists and healthcare experts frequently work together to create customized meal plans that address the unique requirements and difficulties related to the treatment process.

PHYSICAL EXERCISE AND REHABILITATION

During therapy, engaging in physical exercise and rehabilitation is essential. Physical capacities may be limited for individuals based on the type of sickness and recommended therapies. The goals of rehabilitation programs are to increase mobility, improve function, and improve quality of life overall. These programs are meticulously crafted to cater to the distinct requirements of every patient, taking into account variables including the nature of treatment received and its possible influence on physical capabilities. Frequent exercise that is tailored to each person's needs promotes mental health and a sense of normalcy during trying times in addition to helping with physical recuperation.

INTEGRATIVE TREATMENTS FOR COMPLETE WELLNESS

Many people undergoing treatment look at integrative therapies as a complement to traditional medical approaches in their quest for complete well-being. These treatments cover a wide range of techniques, such as massage, acupuncture, mindfulness training, and herbal supplements. The goal of integrating these therapies is to treat the emotional and spiritual elements of sickness in addition to its physical manifestations. While there may be differing degrees of scientific evidence to support some of these therapies, the focus is on offering patients an all-encompassing healing approach that transcends the boundaries of conventional medicine. Integrative therapies frequently provide patients with the tools they need to take an active role in their recovery and improve their general well-being.

Life during treatment is a complex experience that involves navigating the difficulties of dealing with day-to-day issues, taking diet into account, exercising and recovering physically, as well as investigating integrative therapies for overall well-being. Each person's journey is different, and resilience and general wellness can only be fostered through an all-encompassing strategy that takes into account the mental, physical, and spiritual dimensions of health.

CHAPTER FIVE

SURVIVORSHIP AND FUTURE PROSPECTS

LIFE AFTER TREATMENT

For cancer survivors, the period following treatment represents a critical turning point in their journey. Even though the end of treatment is frequently a reason for joy, it also ushers in a phase of transition and acclimatization to a new normal. The psychological and physical effects of cancer and its therapies can have a lasting impact on survivors' outlooks on relationships, life, and personal priorities. Navigating the difficult terrain of survivorship, which includes physical recovery, emotional healing, and reintegration into daily routines, is necessary to embrace life after treatment.

MONITORING AND AFTERCARE

To monitor a patient's health, identify any complications or recurrences, and address the long-term physical and psychological impacts of cancer and its treatments, follow-up care is a crucial part of post-treatment survivorship. Follow-up care is based on routine medical check-ups, imaging investigations, and blood tests. Depending on the type of cancer, diagnosis stage, and personal health concerns, the frequency and severity of these consultations may change. In addition to the physical components, follow-up care frequently involves talking about mental health, changing one's lifestyle, and developing general well-being techniques.

POSSIBLE AFTEREFFECTS AND DIFFICULTIES

A wide range of side effects and issues related to cancer therapies may affect survivors. These may show up months or even years after therapy are over. Physical difficulties like organ failure, hormone abnormalities, or secondary tumors are examples of late impacts. Survivors may also experience mental distress, cognitive problems, and reproduction challenges as late effects. The unpredictable nature of these effects emphasizes how crucial it is for survivors and their healthcare practitioners to stay in constant communication. A comprehensive and customized approach is necessary to comprehend and manage late consequences, taking into account the individuality of each survivor's health profile and experiences.

GETTING BACK TO NORMAL

Following treatment, reintegrating into society is a complex process that includes social reconnection, emotional healing, and physical rehabilitation. Survivors frequently struggle with a variety of feelings, such as thankfulness, worry, and future uncertainty. The process of transitioning involves regaining physical strength through exercise, making healthy lifestyle decisions, and getting emotional assistance from mental health counselors, support groups, or medical specialists. Reestablishing ties with friends, family, and the community is also very important because it creates a network of support that helps with the emotional and social recovery required for a happy life after cancer.

Being a survivor of cancer means going through a complex and dynamic process that doesn't finish with the completion of medical therapy. After treatment, one must adjust to a new normal, manage follow-up care, deal with any aftereffects, and make emotional and social transitions. Healthcare providers can provide individualized support to promote holistic well-being and improve the quality of life for cancer survivors by acknowledging the distinct obstacles they confront.

CHAPTER SIX

ENCOURAGING AND PROVIDING

TAKING UP THE CAUSE OF YOURSELF OR A LOVED ONE

Advocacy is a potent instrument that enables people to express their demands and worries, particularly when confronted with difficult situations like a health emergency. Being an advocate for oneself or a loved one is a life-changing experience that calls for a thorough comprehension of the relevant issues, strong communication abilities, and a readiness to maneuver through intricate systems. Advocacy becomes essential when managing a medical condition such as Ewing Sarcoma to guarantee optimal care and assistance.

One crucial element of self-advocacy is collecting knowledge about the ailment, treatment alternatives, and available resources. Making well-informed decisions entails speaking with medical professionals, doing research, and getting second opinions. It's important to actively participate in the decision-making process, raise concerns, and ask questions to make sure the medical treatment is tailored to the specific needs of the patient.

Being an informed and caring ally is just as important as personally advocating for a loved one who has Ewing Sarcoma. This entails providing emotional support, going to doctor's appointments together, and engaging in dialogue with medical professionals. Being a loved one's voice when needed, making sure their desires are followed, and encouraging open communication between the patient, their medical staff, and other support networks are all components of advocating for a loved one.

INTERACTING WITH THE COMMUNITY FOR EWING SARCOMA

When coping with a unique illness like Ewing Sarcoma, community interaction is a potent approach to finding strength, sharing experiences, and receiving insightful knowledge. Being a member of the Ewing Sarcoma community allows people to interact with others who are cognizant of the particular difficulties they encounter. Social media platforms, online forums, and support groups offer venues for knowledge sharing, personal narrative sharing, and mutual support.

People with Ewing Sarcoma can acquire a feeling of community and learn coping mechanisms that work for other people through community engagement. People can learn from one another, talk about treatment options, and work through the emotional challenges of living with or caring for someone who has Ewing Sarcoma when they share their stories, creating a supportive community.

Moreover, community involvement goes beyond individual assistance to encompass more extensive advocacy. Individuals can support awareness campaigns, fundraising drives, and activities focused on improving research and treatment outcomes by working with groups dedicated to Ewing Sarcoma. The Ewing Sarcoma community's strength as a whole can enhance the effect of advocacy, resulting in greater resources, more awareness, and a more powerful voice in the medical community.

INCREASING CONSCIENCE AND ENDORSING RESEARCH

Increasing public knowledge of Ewing Sarcoma is essential to advocacy because it facilitates early diagnosis, better support for individuals impacted by the condition, and enhanced public understanding of the illness. People may make a big difference in increasing awareness by using social media to reach a wider audience, participating in awareness events, and sharing their stories through various means.

Supporting research is another crucial component of advocacy since it sets the framework for breakthroughs in treatment options and, ultimately, a cure. To further the scientific understanding of Ewing Sarcoma, individuals might work with research organizations, take part in clinical trials, and organize fundraising events. Advocates who actively support research programs are fighting for improved outcomes for the larger community facing comparable issues as well as for themselves or their loved ones.

In the context of Ewing Sarcoma, advocacy and empowerment require a multifaceted strategy. People can have a significant impact on the path of those afflicted by this uncommon and difficult condition by actively participating in research and awareness campaigns, connecting with a supportive network, and advocating for themselves or a loved one.

DEVELOPMENTS IN THE STUDY OF EWING SARCOMA

Research on Ewing sarcoma has advanced significantly throughout time, providing fresh information about this uncommon and severe form of bone cancer and its management. By delving into the disease's molecular nuances, scientists and medical professionals have been able to identify the hereditary foundations of the condition and open the door to more focused treatment strategies. In addition to improving diagnosis accuracy, the discovery of certain genetic abnormalities and molecular pathways linked to Ewing sarcoma has created new opportunities for the development of creative and more successful therapeutic approaches.

Novel technologies, including genome sequencing and sophisticated imaging methods, have been essential in deciphering the intricacies of Ewing sarcoma. With the aid of these instruments, scientists have been able to identify the genetic changes that propel the illness, which has made it easier to create individualized treatment regimens. In addition, cooperative efforts amongst multidisciplinary teams have promoted an all-encompassing strategy for Ewing sarcoma research, uniting specialists in pathology, oncology, and genetics to address the illness from multiple perspectives.

PROSPECTIVE THERAPIES TO COME

The field of treating Ewing sarcoma is changing as a result of the introduction of treatments that show promise for bettering patient outcomes. At the vanguard of these developments are targeted medicines, immunotherapy, and precision medicine techniques, which provide more individualized and efficient options for people with Ewing sarcoma. Scientists are investigating new drugs that target the molecular processes involved in the onset and spread of the disease specifically in an effort to disrupt malignant cells with the least amount of collateral damage to healthy organs.

The ability of immunotherapy in particular to activate the body's immune system to identify and destroy cancer cells has drawn interest. Positive outcomes from early clinical studies investigating immunotherapeutic approaches for Ewing sarcoma have sparked optimism for a paradigm shift in the treatment of this malignancy. Furthermore, improvements in knowledge of the immune system and the tumor microenvironment within Ewing sarcoma lesions are offering important new information for the creation of immunotherapy that work better.

THE IMPACT OF ADVOCACY ON FUTURE DEVELOPMENT

Future directions for the study and therapy of Ewing sarcoma are greatly influenced by advocacy. To expedite research efforts and enhance patient outcomes, patient advocacy groups, nonprofit organizations, and individuals impacted by the disease play a crucial role in generating awareness, organizing resources, and influencing policy. These supporters are strong voices when it comes to encouraging researcher collaboration, pushing for more financing for Ewing sarcoma research, and encouraging the conversion of scientific discoveries into real-world therapeutic advances.

Moreover, advocacy initiatives go beyond the domain of study and care to attend to the comprehensive requirements of those impacted by Ewing sarcoma. Promoting patient-centered treatment, guaranteeing access to high-quality healthcare services, and fighting for laws that enhance patients' and their families' general well-being are all crucial tasks for advocates. Through elevating the voices of those affected by Ewing sarcoma, advocates play a vital role in fostering a more empathetic and supportive environment that enables people to overcome the obstacles posed by the illness.